GOD WILL HEAL EVEN THE WORST SINNERS OF ANY SICKNESS

Amb. Promise Ogbonna

CONTENTS

Why I Wrote This Book!

The Heavenly Mandate & Vision

First Words

Chapter 1 His Healing Is for The World; His Health Is for Christ Ambassadors

Chapter 2 Healing is for The Whole Man

Chapter 3 What Causes Unbelief and What Enforces Faith

Chapter 4 Created to Do Good Works - Healing All

Chapter 5 Never Touch All Jesus Carried.

Chapter 6 Proclaim Liberty to The Captives

Chapter 7 Medicine and Physicians

Chapter 8 The Door to The Miraculous

Chapter 9 God's ordained Way to a Healthy Life

Become a Citizen of Heaven Today

About the Author-Amb Promise Ogbonna

Other Books by The Author

Connect with The Author

Our Healing Products

Our Special Services

WHY I WROTE THIS BOOK!

I am sent to Publish All the Words of God's Heavenly Kingdom Life for the Restoration of all.

I am not writing human philosophy. I am not writing as a hobby neither am I writing to entertain but to bring Spiritual light, impart Spiritual Wisdom and Power to build your faith and transform your life! I have a Mandate from The Lord Jesus Christ to write and these Words are published to meet man's needs in every area of life! This Book, therefore, is published in obedience to the Command of the Lord to make His Words of Life and Wisdom Solutions and Power available to address every aspect of human needs.

I can say as Paul wrote "My message and my preaching were not in the persuasive language of philosophy, but in demonstration of the Spirit and of power; in order that your faith should rest, not on human philosophy, but on the power of God." 1 Corinthians 2:4-5 (BBE)

"For the Kingdom of God is based, not on words, but on power." 1 Corinthians 4:20 (BBE)

The Life Publishing Mandate

The Lord sent me to Publish All the Words of His Heavenly Kingdom Life for ALL mankind!

Jesus' last words is to Preach and Publish the Goodnews with proofs to every creature and among all nations (Mark 13:10; 16:15; Matthew 24:14).

The Lord gave us the Goodnews to publish and spread among all nations (Psalm 68:11; Mark 13:10).

In the Book of Esther, the enemy wrote and spread the words of death worldwide to destroy God's people and souls that God loves. [see Esther 3].

But at the command of the king, a new decree and words of life were written and spread to reach everyone (every creature) everywhere that the first words of death had reached. [see Esther 8].

This is our task. We have been given the New Covenant, Heavenly Kingdom, Words of Life to publish and spread to reach every creature everywhere worldwide. The Goodnews is that no one needs to die again! The old decree has been changed. Everyone can now live and enjoy peace and prosperity where each lives. That is why Ontop Mission Life Publishers Company. We are Publishing, Spreading and Bringing the Gospel of Christ and All the Words of life to every creature everywhere.

I would like to share some of the encounters with the Lord Jesus Christ that gave birth to The Life Publishing Mandate and why this Book and my other books:

1. On 21or5or95, Jesus Christ and I stood on the balcony of a great beautiful mansion in Heaven whose foundation I couldn't see (see Amos 9:6). He showed me Preachers, driven by selfishness and being used by the enemy, walking on people's heads and shoulders as their platform to preach. The people were hungry, thirsty, weeping, trampled upon and yet yearning for the TRUTH (see Amos 8:11-13). I saw My Lord shaking His head in disgust. He also brought to my view those in hell and I saw their agony and pain and what a sight it was! Afterward, as we beheld the abuse of His people, He pointed His right hand towards them and said to me, "See what is happening to the people I died for. "The Lord Jesus gave me A WELL USED COPY OF THE BIBLE and said to me "GO and tell them (The Preachers and The People) to Repent and Believe the Gospel Only and they will be Restored." I asked 'How

will I do it? And He said to me, "BE SEPARATE! Go, I send YOU as My Ambassador and Witness with My Authority and Power: Publish the Word, stop anything after their destruction, Raise, Build and Plant them as My Ambassadors. Let them know the truth. Teach All the TRUTH and Spread them as My Seed ALL over the earth and restore all things."

2. On 6or7or96, The Lord Jesus Christ came to me again and said, "It is well" and gave me a copy of THE BIBLE and said to me, "Take: This is My Staff of Office" – My Authority and Power. After The LORD gave me His Staff of Office [The Word], I saw something like a mist or cloud appear out of the Word and as I watched, a horse emerged from 'within the mist' and jumped about and stopped. The Lord told me The Word is creative and created the horse and is My Rod for working Miracles, Wonders and Signs. I am to Go with it to all, as Moses went with his ROD, and "Stop anything after man's destruction, Bring Healing, Liberty and Restoration to all; Raise, Build and Plant Christ's Ambassadors everywhere and Restore all things."

3. On 20or5or97, I was given a BIBLE and 2 BIROS by Arch. Benson A. Idahosa in a conference that took place in a place like a stadium. And he said to me, "Go and Proclaim and Publish the Everlasting Gospel of Jesus Christ worldwide and deliver the full benefits to all. This Gospel of The Kingdom must be preached in all the world for a witness unto all nations!

4. On 18or11or03, The Lord spoke to me again ON WRITING, and said to me "Write all the hidden mysteries I show you and I will ensure it gets to all the Nations Prophetic writings is what unveils, reveals, makes known the revelation of the mystery hidden for ages long past. The surest way of unveiling the Gospel and proclaim Jesus Christ the Lord is through prophetic writings as God commanded so that all nations will believe and obey God.

5. On 26or11or03, The Lord spoke to me saying, "Write what people can read and understand. It's most important. Your writing must be readable and understandable. Write in such a way that a primary school pupil can read and understand My Words. "The common people heard me gladly." Everyone must read and

understand My Words that you write.

6. On 2or10or04, The Lord Jesus explained to me the vision of 21or5or95 where I Stood with Him on the Balcony of the Mansion in Heaven and He showed me Preachers using the shoulders and heads of people as their platform to preach. They were hungry, thirsty and trampled underfoot yet yearning for the reality. And The Lord commanded me to WRITE and publish His Words for the downtrodden and for all."

7. On10or12or04, The Lord said to me "Write in a book all the Words that I have spoken to you" and He gave me Jeremiah 30:2.

8. On 04or04or05, The Lord said to me "Publish the Word and bring healing, liberty and restoration to all everywhere." See Psalm 68:11 and Psalm 107:20.

9. On 23or12or05, The Lord said to me:
Publish the Words
Publish the Works
Publish the Wonders
Make My Deeds Known
Let Everyone See My Glory Everywhere
10. On 01or03or13, The Holy Ghost said to me:
Publish the Works of Jesus Christ everywhere
Advertise the Doings of Jesus Christ the Lord.
Make known the Miracles of Jesus Christ the Lord.
Bind the Testimony of the Acts of the Lord Jesus Christ.
Be My Witness of all My Signs and Wonders everywhere.
Share Testimonies of All I AM Doing forever.
Go and Tell All everywhere of All My Miracles and Wonders and Signs and All I have Done and Commanded you.

The Lord said to me "All who believe that I sent you and receive you as My Ambassador and receive your Words as My Words will experience all the Father sent me to make available to humanity!"

Like Peter, I can tell you "We have not followed cunningly devised fables, when we made known unto you the power and coming of our Lord Jesus Christ, but were eyewitnesses of his majesty." 2Peter 1:16

Beloved, every Word written in this Book is from The Lord and are His Wisdom and Heaven's Solutions packaged and released to deal with your challenges, solve your problems and meet your needs.

Read with an open heart, Believe and Receive the Truth and Pick the Lessons and engage them.

I know you will experience The One who is The Author, Perfecter and Finisher of your faith and Who is The Real Author of this Book. He is Jesus Christ, The Son of The Living God. And He is the Same yesterday and today and forever!

"O LORD, how manifold are Your works! In wisdom You have made them all. The earth is full of Your possessions." Psalm 104:24

I guarantee you that you will never be the same again as you embrace God's Wisdom in This Book!

God Bless you.

Your Brother and His Steward for the benefit of all,

Ambassador Promise Ogbonna

THE HEAVENLY MANDATE & VISION

The Heavenly Mandate

To Preach the Everlasting Gospel to Everyone everywhere, stop anything after man's destruction, Bring Healing, Liberty and Restoration to ALL; Raise, Build and Plant All as Christ's Ambassadors on His Living Mission everywhere and Restore all things!

The Heavenly Vision

To Restore All Things Everywhere at All Cost and By All Means! Acts 3:21

FIRSTWORDS

There is no excuse why anyone who is sick should remain sick. There is no reason why everyone sick today should not be healed no matter the cause of the sickness or disease.

Sickness is not the Will of God for anyone! Never forever.

God's wish above all else is for everyone diseased and sick to be healed and be in health.

And God has done all that is required for all the sick to be healed and set free from every sickness and disease.

Listen to this: He that commits sin is of the devil; for the devil sinned from the beginning. For this purpose, the Son of God was manifested, that he might destroy the works of the devil.

The truth is that Jesus Christ came to destroy the works of the devil and unless and until He does destroy the works of the devil, He cannot be said to have succeeded in His Mission and Mandate. Sin and Sickness are the works of the devil and Jesus must destroy both!

Therefore, "God anointed Jesus of Nazareth with the Holy Spirit and with power, who went about doing good and healing ALL who were oppressed by the devil, for God was with Him."

This Book 'God Will Heal Even the Worst Sinners of Any Sickness' points every sick person to the provisions of God for the Healing of everyone – even the worst sinners!

Yes, there are people whose sins are responsible for their sicknesses. Notwithstanding, there is no justifiable reason why ANY sin should hinder the Healing of anyone who is sick today!

No matter your sins, the full price has been paid for your healing to be enforced.

Yes "God Will Heal Even the Worst Sinners of Any Sickness!" And this Book shows how.

Read with an open heart and Rise and take your healing by the force of Faith today!

Peace in Jesus Almighty Healing name!

CHAPTER 1

*His Healing Is for The World; His
Health Is for Christ Ambassadors*

Under the Old Covenant, Israel walked in health whenever they obeyed God's commands and kept His Statutes. Walking in line with God's word was all Israel needed to walk in God's health.

Healing was God's provision for all who disobeyed God and become victims and prisoners to sickness and disease.

Numbers 21:1-9 (Let us Read and Note what it says)

1 The king of Arad, the Canaanite, who dwelt in the South, heard that Israel was coming on the road to Atari, then he fought against Israel and took some of them prisoners.

2 So Israel made a vow to the LORD, and said, "If You will indeed deliver this people into my hand, then I will utterly destroy their cities."

3 And the LORD listened to the voice of Israel and delivered up the Canaanites, and they utterly destroyed them and their cities. So the name of that place was called Hormah.

4 Then they journeyed from Mount Hor by the Way of the Red Sea, to go around the land of Edom; and the soul of the people became very discouraged on the way.

5 And the people spoke against God and against Moses: "Why have you brought us up out of Egypt to die in the wilderness? For

there is no food and no water, and our soul loathes this worthless bread."

6 So the LORD sent fiery serpents among the people, and they bit the people; and many of the people of Israel died.

7 Therefore the people came to Moses, and said, "We have sinned, for we have spoken against the LORD and against you; pray to the LORD that He take away the serpents from us." So Moses prayed for the people.

8 Then the LORD said to Moses, "Make a fiery serpent, and set it on a pole; and it shall be that everyone who is bitten, when he looks at it, shall live."

9 So Moses made a bronze serpent, and put it on a pole; and so it was, if a serpent had bitten anyone, when he looked at the bronze serpent, he lived.

Until Israel sinned, and became vulnerable to the serpents' attack, not one of them was bitten by the serpent. Even as the serpent was having a field day, Joshua and Caleb and their household were preserved from that plague because they kept God's commands and statutes and fully followed the LORD with a perfect heart. No harm befell them. You can be kept as they were. All it takes is total commitment to obeying the word of the LORD and His commands. Health is for obedient and committed followers.

Healing was God's provision for fallen Israelites.

That means, anytime any Israelite disobeyed God's word and was attacked by sickness or disease; God made available His healing to the repentant Israelite.

Jesus went about – doing good and healing all – in order to fulfill the Old Testament or Covenant or Law and Prophets.

God's healing power was made available to the Jews or Israel.

Note – Romans 2:28-29, Romans 9:6-8; Galatians 6:16, Galatians 3:26-29.

Romans 2:28-29 says "For he is not a Jew who is one outwardly, nor is circumcision that which is outward in the flesh; but he is a Jew who is one inwardly; and circumcision is that of the heart, in the Spirit, not in the letter; whose praise is not from men but from God."

Romans 9:6-8 says "But it is not that the word of God has taken no effect. For they are not all Israel who are of Israel, nor are they all children because they are the seed of Abraham; but, "In Isaac your seed shall be called. That is, those who are the children of the flesh, these are not the children of God; but the children of the promise are counted as the seed."

Galatians 6:15-16 "For in Christ Jesus neither circumcision nor uncircumcision avails anything, but a new creation. And as many as walk according to this rule, peace and mercy be upon them, and upon the Israel of God."

Now hear this amazing revelation in Galatians 3:22-4:7:

22 But the Scripture has confined all under sin, that the promise by faith in Jesus Christ might be given to those who believe.

23 But before faith came, we were kept under guard by the law, kept for the faith which would afterward be revealed.

24 Therefore the law was our tutor to bring us to Christ, that we might be justified by faith.

25 But after faith has come, we are no longer under a tutor.

26 For you are all sons of God through faith in Christ Jesus.

27 For as many of you as were baptized into Christ have put on Christ.

28 There is neither Jew nor Greek, there is neither slave nor free, there is neither male nor female; for you are all one in Christ Jesus.

29 And if you are Christ's, then you are Abraham's seed, and heirs according to the promise.

Galatians 4:1-7

1 ¶ Now I say that the heir, as long as he is a child, does not differ at all from a slave, though he is master of all,

2 but is under guardians and stewards until the time appointed by the father.

3 Even so we, when we were children, were in bondage under the elements of the world.

4 But when the fullness of the time had come, God sent forth His Son, born of a woman, born under the law,

5 to redeem those who were under the law, that we might re-

ceive the adoption as sons.

6 And because you are sons, God has sent forth the Spirit of His Son into your hearts, crying out, "Abba, Father!"

7 Therefore you are no longer a slave but a son, and if a son, then an heir of God through Christ.

HALLELUYAH!!!

I am God's Heir now! In Christ Jesus I am God's Son in Christ's very class. And so are you if you are born again.

That means all the Father owns on earth are ours. The Kingdom, the power, the glory and all things are now ours as God them all to Adam in the beginning and as He restored all to Christ after his resurrection.

The reason for the suffering of the body of Christ is her ignorance.

It is written in Isaiah 5:13 "Therefore, my people have gone into captivity, because they have no knowledge; Their honorable men are famished, and their multitude dried up with thirst."

God says Hosea 4:6 "My people are destroyed for lack of knowledge. Because you have rejected knowledge, I also will reject you from being priest for Me; Because you have forgotten the law of your God, I also will forget your children."

Psalms 82:5-7 says:

5 They do not know, nor do they understand; They walk about in darkness; All the foundations of the earth are unstable.

6 I said, "You are gods, and all of you are children of the Highest.

7 But you shall die like men, and fall like one of the princes."

Healing is God's provision to restore His Children to what they were entitled to by obeying God's word or if they had kept the covenant.

Therefore, healing is God's provision for all those who had defaulted the covenant and became victims as a result.

Health is the entitlement of all covenant practitioners.

But Healing is God's provision to restore all covenant defaulters to their entitlement of health.

God sent His word and healed them, and delivered them from their destructions.

In one word, God's word served as a PRESERVATIVE.

Psalms 107:20 He sent His word and healed them, and delivered them from their destructions.

The Word is life to those who find it and health to all their flesh. Proverbs 4:20-22

20 My son, give attention to my words; Incline your ear to my sayings.

21 Do not let them depart from your eyes; Keep them in the midst of your heart;

22 For they are life to those who find them, And health to all their flesh.

Through the Word, our souls are preserved, we are persevered from all evil; our going out and our coming in is preserved. The LORD preserves those who obey His word, keep His commands or hearken to His Statutes.

Psalms 121:7-8

7 The LORD shall preserve you from all evil; He shall preserve your soul.

8 The LORD shall preserve your going out and your coming in from this time forth, and even forevermore.

Jesus came as the word made flesh

John 1:1, 14

1 In the beginning was the Word, and the Word was with God, and the Word was God.

14 And the Word became flesh and dwelt among us, and we beheld His glory, the glory as of the only begotten of the Father, full of grace and truth.

And as many as touched him were made well whole

Mark 6:56

Wherever He entered into villages, cities, or in the country, they laid the sick in the marketplaces, and begged Him that they might just touch the hem of His garment. And as many as touched Him were made well.

Why did He come?

·To fulfill the Old Covenant.

·To destroy the wall of partition so that all can come back to

God.

•To save the whole world- The lost.

Healing, He said is the Children's bread

Mark 7:27

But Jesus said to her, "Let the children be filled first, for it is not good to take the children's bread and throw it to the little dogs."

He healed Abraham's daughter whom Satan bound

Luke 13:10-16

10 Now He was teaching in one of the synagogues on the Sabbath.

11 And behold, there was a woman who had a spirit of infirmity eighteen years, and was bent over and could in no way raise herself up.

12 But when Jesus saw her, He called her to Him and said to her, "Woman, you are loosed from your infirmity."

13 And He laid His hands on her, and immediately she was made straight, and glorified God.

14 But the ruler of the synagogue answered with indignation, because Jesus had healed on the Sabbath; and he said to the crowd, "There are six days on which men ought to work; therefore come and be healed on them, and not on the Sabbath day."

15 The Lord then answered him and said, "Hypocrite! Does not each one of you on the Sabbath loose his ox or donkey from the stall, and lead it away to water it?

16 "So ought not this woman, being a daughter of Abraham, whom Satan has bound for eighteen years, be loosed from this bond on the Sabbath?"

Acts 10:38

How God anointed Jesus of Nazareth with the Holy Spirit and with power, who went about doing good and healing all who were oppressed by the devil, for God was with Him.

He refused to heal the woman of Canaan's daughter but was compelled to do so when He saw her great faith

Mathew 15:22-28

22 And behold, a woman of Canaan came from that region and cried out to Him, saying, "Have mercy on me, O Lord, Son of

David! My daughter is severely demon-possessed."

23 But He answered her not a word. And His disciples came and urged Him, saying, "Send her away, for she cries out after us."

24 But He answered and said, "I was not sent except to the lost sheep of the house of Israel."

25 Then she came and worshiped Him, saying, "Lord, help me!"

26 But He answered and said, "It is not good to take the children's bread and throw it to the little dogs."

27 And she said, "Yes, Lord, yet even the little dogs eat the crumbs which fall from their masters' table."

28 Then Jesus answered and said to her, "O woman, great is your faith! Let it be to you as you desire." And her daughter was healed from that very hour.

It was the Children's right legally to be healed because the devil is the one who has bound them and is oppressing them. We are God's children. We are also Abraham's children. So if Jesus loosed the daughter (child) of Abraham whom Satan bound, would He not heal all bound and oppressed by Satan who are not only Abraham's children (See Galatians 3:26-29), but God's children (see 2 Corinthians 6:16-18; Galatians 4:1-7; Romans 8:14-17)

Galatians 3:26-29

26 For you are all sons of God through faith in Christ Jesus.

27 For as many of you as were baptized into Christ have put on Christ.

28 There is neither Jew nor Greek, there is neither slave nor free, there is neither male nor female; for you are all one in Christ Jesus.

29 And if you are Christ's, then you are Abraham's seed, and heirs according to the promise.

No-one who Satan has bound and oppressing with sickness must be left in Satan's bondage.

If Jesus went about doing good and healing all of Abraham's children whom Satan kept in bondage and oppression, then because He is the Lord and cannot change, the same always (Exodus 3:14, Malachi 3:6; Exodus 15:26; 23:25-26; Hebrews 13:8), He still will heal all Abraham's Children whom Satan has bound and are being oppressed .

Above all, He cannot leave any of God's children under Satan's bondage and oppression.

This is why All who are bound (Romans 8:19-23) must be loosed and set free by The Lord (Luke 4:18:19, Acts 10:38)

Destroy Satan's work

1 John 3:8

He who sins is of the devil, for the devil has sinned from the beginning. For this purpose the Son of God was manifested, that He might destroy the works of the devil

Acts 10:38

How God anointed Jesus of Nazareth with the Holy Spirit and with power, who went about doing good and healing all who were oppressed by the devil, for God was with Him.

John 14:12

Most assuredly, I say to you, he who believes in Me, the works that I do he will do also; and greater works than these he will do, because I go to My Father.

Proverbs 13:17

A wicked messenger falls into trouble, but a faithful ambassador brings health.

Everyone in the world who is sick is qualified for healing because they are under Satanic captivity just as the Israelites were when they fell out of God's favour because of sin (Numbers 21:7-9; John 3:14-18, 36)

Satan hath bound Abraham's daughter

Luke 13:10-16

10 Now He was teaching in one of the synagogues on the Sabbath.

11 And behold, there was a woman who had a spirit of infirmity eighteen years, and was bent over and could in no way raise herself up.

12 But when Jesus saw her, He called her to Him and said to her, "Woman, you are loosed from your infirmity."

13 And He laid His hands on her, and immediately she was made straight, and glorified God.

14 But the ruler of the synagogue answered with indignation, because Jesus had healed on the Sabbath; and he said to the crowd, "There are six days on which men ought to work; therefore come and be healed on them, and not on the Sabbath day."

15 The Lord then answered him and said, "Hypocrite! Does not each one of you on the Sabbath loose his ox or donkey from the stall, and lead it away to water it?

16 "So ought not this woman, being a daughter of Abraham, whom Satan has bound for eighteen years, be loosed from this bond on the Sabbath?"

Acts 10:38

How God anointed Jesus of Nazareth with the Holy Spirit and with power, who went about doing good and healing all who were oppressed by the devil, for God was with Him.

Satan hath bound mankind

Romans 8:19-23

19 For the earnest expectation of the creation eagerly waits for the revealing of the sons of God.

20 For the creation was subjected to futility, not willingly, but because of Him who subjected it in hope;

21 Because the creation itself also will be delivered from the bondage of corruption into the glorious liberty of the children of God.

22 For we know that the whole creation groans and labors with birth pangs together until now.

23 Not only that, but we also who have the first fruits of the Spirit, even we ourselves groan within ourselves, eagerly waiting for the adoption, the redemption of our body.

Acts 10:38

How God anointed Jesus of Nazareth with the Holy Spirit and with power, who went about doing good and healing all who were oppressed by the devil, for God was with Him.

If Christ loosed Abraham's daughter, there is no excuse why He will not lose all under satanic bounds today.

Healing still remains the children's bread (Mark 7:27)

And by faith, the dogs can take the crumbs and be healed. So, none will be abandoned in his or her sickness!

Faith has bridged the gap. To whoever believes, all things (even healing) is possible. (Mark 9:23).

Healing is God's provision to restore us to health.

John 10:10

The thief does not come except to steal, and to kill, and to destroy. I have come that they may have life, and that they may have it more abundantly.

Jesus came to give us life totally so that we can live once more and enjoy God's health.

Healing is the Children's bread. Rescue the Bread.

Health is the Son's life. Enjoy the life.

Note: before His death, Jesus went everywhere healing the sick and all who were under the oppression of the devil. He healed all.

On the cross, Jesus took our sins

1 Peter 2:24

Who Himself bore our sins in His own body on the tree, that we, having died to sins, might live for righteousness--by whose stripes you were healed.

On the cross, Jesus took our sicknesses or diseases

Mathew 8:17

That it might be fulfilled which was spoken by Isaiah the prophet, saying: "He Himself took our infirmities and bore our sicknesses."

On the cross, Jesus ended all sicknesses or diseases

Isaiah 53:4-5

4 Surely, He has borne our griefs and carried our sorrows; Yet we esteemed Him stricken, Smitten by God, and afflicted.

5 But He was wounded for our transgressions, He was bruised for our iniquities; The chastisement for our peace was upon Him, And by His stripes we are healed.

Mathew 8:17

That it might be fulfilled which was spoken by Isaiah the prophet, saying: "He Himself took our infirmities and bore our sicknesses."

1 Peter 2:24

Who Himself bore our sins in His own body on the tree, that we, having died to sins, might live for righteousness--by whose stripes you were healed.

Galatians 3:13-14

13 Christ has redeemed us from the curse of the law, having become a curse for us (for it is written, "Cursed is everyone who hangs on a tree"),

14 That the blessing of Abraham might come upon the Gentiles in Christ Jesus, that we might receive the promise of the Spirit through faith.

Now that the cross is past, sin is past, sickness is past; Disease is past. Death is past. Poverty is ended. Curses are ended.

Unless the believer allows it, sickness or disease etc cannot touch us "We have been healed" "We were healed"

He took our sickness in His body. There is nothing left for us to take. Unless we allow or permit the devil to put sickness into our lives, we cannot be sick. Jesus took our diseases away. We have none to take today unless we allow Satan to put on us what is not ours.

After the resurrection, none of Christ's disciples was sick. Jesus is in us now. He is not sick. He is God's life or health.

He is in us in His resurrected state and so we now represent Him.

We are here as His Health Advertisers- advertising His Health where man is found.

We are living epistles (2 Corinthians 3:3) glorifying Him in our bodies (1 Corinthians 6:20)

We have Christ life made manifest in our bodies (2 Corinthians 4:10-11 Amplified).

God's final will is that we BE IN HEALTH. Completely showing forth His life, health and power.

Walk in His Health. Take His Word and Enjoy His life and health

Proverbs 20:22

Do not say, "I will recompense evil"; Wait for the LORD, and He will save you.

CHAPTER 2

John 7 21:23 (NIV)

21Jesus said to them, "I did one miracle, and you are all astonished.

22 Yet because Moses gave you circumcision (though actually it is come from Moses, but from the Patriarchs), and you circumcise a child on the Sabbath.

23 Now If a child can be circumcision on the Sabbath, so that the law of Moses may not be broken, why are you angry with Me for HEALING THE MAN ON THE SABBAT (See John 5:1-14)

Note: Jesus HEALED THE WHOLE MAN.

Isn't that amazing? After He healed the man, no trace of sickness, disease, bodily affliction, infirmity or anything that constitutes the whole man- SPIRIT, SOUL & BODY. It was the whole man Jesus healed.

Jesus has not changed. He is still in that same business of His. He still heals the whole man today as He did before. And He will never stop doing such good work and healing all who are oppressed of the devil. That is God's job descriptions for Jesus forever (Acts 10:38, 1 John 3:8)

His Word is settled in Heaven forever.

Psalms 119:89

Forever, O LORD, Your word is settled in heaven.

He sent- His settled and healed them and delivered them from their destructions.

Psalms 107:20

He sent His word and healed them, and delivered them from their destructions.

Acts 10:38

How God anointed Jesus of Nazareth with the Holy Spirit and with power, who went about doing good and healing all who were oppressed by the devil, for God was with Him.

For this purpose the Son of God was manifested, that He might destroy the works of the devil.

1 John 3:8;

He who sins is of the devil, for the devil has sinned from the beginning. For this purpose the Son of God was manifested, that He might destroy the works of the devil

Hebrews 13:8;

Jesus Christ, the same yesterday, and today, and FOREVER.

Jesus is the same forever. And His Job description is the same forever. Therefore He will not stop doing good and healing all who are oppressed of the devil forever.

Man may change. But He cannot change. He will do His work even if man thinks otherwise.

He is here to heal the whole man- spirit, and soul and body. Whatever is your need, today and now is your time of appointment. He is more than willing to heal you. Are you ready? He will heal you if only you believe.

CHAPTER 3

Signs, Wonders, Miracles, Great and Mighty Deeds Are What We Need to Compel the World to Believe in Our Gospel and Accept Jesus Our Master as Their Saviour And Lord!

Luke 24:11 (New Life Version)

Their words sounded like foolish talk (fairy tales or stories) the followers did not believe them.

The truth about Christ's Virgin birth, His resurrection, His being God, though born as a man, his deity, His being alive today as Christ, The Holy Spirit, sounds like foolish talk, fairly tales, stories that are idle, cock and bull stories to the hearers. The result is that they don't believe in Him (See 1 Corinthians 1 18-25 (NIV)).

The massage of Christ's death on a cross to save man from sins is hard for the religious (Jews) to believe while the Greeks (Thinkers, Philosophers or Educated or Learned) think it is foolish.

God's plan looked foolish to men, but it is wiser than the best plans of men. God's plan which may look weak is stronger than the strongest plan of men in accomplishing result.

Those who are walking in unbelief are those who have chosen

to disbelieve the word of life they have heard.

What can be done to compel them to believe? Give them the evidence that validates the massage.

John 20:6-8;

6 Then Simon Peter came, following him, and went into the tomb; and he saw the linen cloths lying there,

7 And the handkerchief that had been around His head, not lying with the linen cloths, but folded together in a place by itself.

8 Then the other disciple, who came to the tomb first, went in also; and he saw and believed.

John 2:11, 23;

11 This beginning of signs Jesus did in Cana of Galilee, and manifested His glory; and His disciples believed in Him.

23 Now when He was in Jerusalem at the Passover, during the feast, many believed in His name when they saw the signs which He did.

Unless they see, they cannot believe-

John 4: 48;

Then Jesus said to him, "Unless you people see signs and wonders, you will by no means believe."

What causes unbelief is hearing words without proofs, signs and wonders. Those that lived in Christ's time questioned him. Their question is still the question of the entire world of unbelievers.

John 6:30 captures it for us.

"So, they asked Him, "What miraculous signs then will You give, that we may SEE it and BELIEVE You?

Signs, Wonders, Miracles, Great or Mighty Deeds Are What We Need to Compel the World to Believe in Our Gospel and Accept Jesus Christ.

Therefore, to compel and enforce faith in them, do miraculous signs and wonders as Jesus did.

John 14:12;

Those who believe, the same works that I do he shall they do also; greater works or miracles, signs and wonders than these that

I do, shall they do

Jesus did great miracles, signs, wonders.

Acts 10:38

How God anointed Jesus of Nazareth with the Holy Spirit and with power, who went about doing good and healing all who were oppressed by the devil, for God was with Him.

(see Mathew 4:23-25; 9:35; John 6:1-2, 14-15; John 11:45; John 7:31; John 10:32, 41, 42; 25:37-38; John 12:9-11, 42; John 12 17-21; John 20:30-31; 21:25; John 4:45-53; Mark 3:7-8, 10-11 etc)

Wonders, Miracles, Signs, the living proofs and mighty deeds are a must if unbelief in both the Jews and the Greeks (Religious or Educated ones) must be erased and eradicated and bring them to faith.

Please Note: Signs, wonders, Miracles, great and mighty deeds are what we need today to compel everyone - both the religious and the thinking educated one (all unbelievers in the word) to believe in our Gospel and accept our master Jesus as their Saviour, and Lord and Master, too.

This is why we must seek God and His Holy Spirit and Empowerment so that we can reproduce the mighty deeds Jesus and the early apostles did in their time. (See Acts 2:22, Hebrews 2:4; 2 Corinthians 12:12; Romans 15:19-20; Acts 4:30, 5:12-16; 8:6-13; 9:32-48; 19:11-12, 20; Acts 28:8-9)

No one, no matter how unbelieving and hard-hearted will see incredible Signs, Miracles, Wonders, Great Mighty deeds of God and still remain adamant to the Gospel. They must turn to see these great sights.

Even Moses could not be attracted to God until he saw a living sign or miracles that compelled him to wonder. (See the Story in Exodus 3:1- 4, 17).

Moses "SAW" before he was compelled to go over and SEE more of this strange sight- the wonder of why the bush did not burn up. (Exodus 3:3). God had to use a sign and wonder to draw even Moses to himself. (He has used Signs and Wonders to draw many other Ministers including me)

"Unless they see miraculous signs and wonders, they will

NEVER believe" is God's verdict. Therefore, to compel them to believe, God had to use miraculous signs, wonders, great or mighty deeds.

And of God did so, Christ did so, the apostles did so, Paul did so, You and I must NEVER desire to do less. We must do so.

Talk is cheap. Everyone can speak. All may preach. Many may teach. But all these and more will never compel the world to believe. Only signs, wonders, miracles, Great or mighty deeds will compel them to believe and accept the gospel and our saviour and Lord and Master- Jesus Christ.

Don't belittle the power of signs and wonders. Don't speak or teach or preach against signs and wonders.

God wants all to come back to him. Signs or wonders or living miracles are His tools to bring them to Himself to Hear Him.

Do as Jesus did. Do signs. Do miracles. Do wonders. Do great or mighty deeds.

Proverbs 14:28 (NIV)

A large population is king's glory, but without people a prince is ruined (Please take note of this scripture).

The king may be the most powerful and have all the kingdom. But without a large population, the king is reduced to nothing and will be ruined.

A large population is the King's glory. A small population is the King's shame, reproach and destruction or downfall.

Without subjects, a prince is ruined. But with subject, the king is preserved and the kingdom kept safe.

There is much the church can do once the population of the church increases more than the opposition (or unbelievers).

When the church commands more in population, then she will become the decision maker in all affairs of the world. The enemy understands this and so is all out to stop the growth of the church.

The Devil's method is to stop by all means and at all cost the growth of the church by ensuring that miracles, signs and wonders are no longer done in the church. For he knows, if signs, wonders, miracles do not happen, to increase the population of the church will be very difficult. More so, adopting other means of church growth will mean the spending of funds or money and resources which could have been used to reach more with the healing power of God.

And until you can reach them, you can't do anything for them- the unreached

Whatever can stop signs and wonders can stop the growth of the church and this would mean the dominion of Satan via his more population worshippers and children over the church.

Go for God's Best. Go for signs, wonders and miracles. It is the only tool and the most efficient and effective means ordained by God to increase the population of His church and rule the world.

Be fruitful, Increase, multiply; Replenish the earth, subdue it; and have dominion over all.

Genesis 1:28;

Then God blessed them, and God said to them, "Be fruitful and multiply; fill the earth and subdue it; have dominion over the fish of the sea, over the birds of the air, and over every living thing that moves on the earth."

To do so, we must take over the population of the world. And to take over the world's population, we must do signs, wonders, miracles and mighty deeds.

CHAPTER 4

*CREATED TO DO GOOD
WORKS - HEALING ALL*

"**G**od Anointed Jesus Christ with the Holy Ghost and with power and he went about doing good and healing all who were oppressed of the devil; for God was with him" (Acts 10:38). Compare with Ephesians 2:10 (NIV).

"For we are God's workmanship, created in Christ Jesus to do GOOD WORKS (and heal all who are oppressed of the devil), which God prepared in advance for us TO DO (Good works and HEAL ALL who are oppressed of the devil).

Ephesians 3:10-11 (NIV)

10 His intent was that NOW, through the Church, the manifold wisdom of God (ways of God) should be made known to the ruler and authorities in the heavenly places,

11 according to HIS ETERNAL PURPOSE WHICH HE (GOD) ACCOMPLISHED IN CHRIST JESUS OUR LORD,

What Is God's Eternal Purpose Which He God Accomplished in Christ Jesus Our Lord?

3 John 2

Beloved, I pray that you may prosper in all things and be in health, just as your soul prospers.

1 John 3:8

He who sins is of the devil, for the devil has sinned from the beginning. For this purpose the Son of God was manifested, that He might destroy the works of the devil.

Acts 10:38

How God anointed Jesus of Nazareth with the Holy Spirit and with power, who went about doing good and healing all who were oppressed by the devil, for God was with Him.

John 3:14-18

14 And as Moses lifted up the serpent in the wilderness, even so must the Son of Man be lifted up,

15 That whoever believes in Him should not perish but have eternal life.

16 For God so loved the world that He gave His only begotten Son, that whoever believes in Him should not perish but have everlasting life.

17 For God did not send His Son into the world to condemn the world, but that the world through Him might be saved.

18 He who believes in Him is not condemned; but he who does not believe is condemned already, because he has not believed in the name of the only begotten Son of God.

Luke 4:18-19. 40-41

18 The Spirit of the LORD is upon Me, Because He has anointed Me To preach the gospel to the poor; He has sent Me to heal the brokenhearted, to proclaim liberty to the captives and recovery of sight to the blind, to set at liberty those who are oppressed;

19 To proclaim the acceptable year of the LORD."

40 When the sun was setting, all those who had any that were sick with various diseases brought them to Him; and He laid His hands on every one of them and healed them.

41 And demons also came out of many, crying out and saying, "You are the Christ, the Son of God!" And He, rebuking them, did not allow them to speak, for they knew that He was the Christ.

Luke 13:10-16

10 Now He was teaching in one of the synagogues on the Sabbath.

11 And behold, there was a woman who had a spirit of infirmity

eighteen years, and was bent over and could in no way raise herself up.

12 But when Jesus saw her, He called her to Him and said to her, "Woman, you are loosed from your infirmity."

13 And He laid His hands on her, and immediately she was made straight, and glorified God.

14 But the ruler of the synagogue answered with indignation, because Jesus had healed on the Sabbath; and he said to the crowd, "There are six days on which men ought to work; therefore come and be healed on them, and not on the Sabbath day."

15 The Lord then answered him and said, "Hypocrite! Does not each one of you on the Sabbath loose his ox or donkey from the stall, and lead it away to water it?

16 "So ought not this woman, being a daughter of Abraham, whom Satan has bound--think of it--for eighteen years, be loosed from this bond on the Sabbath?"

Man's eternal salvation (redemption) from sin and all of its consequences and man's exaltation as God's to rule and dominate the earth as God the heavens (Psalms 115:16; psalms 8:3-6, psalms 82:6; Genesis 1:26-28) has been and still remains God's ultimate plan.

For God to Accomplish this His eternal purpose, what did He do?

He made us ONE in Christ and with Christ.

Ephesians 2:11-22

11 Formerly you who are Gentiles by birth as called "Uncircumcised"

12 At one time you were separated from Christ, exclusive from citizenship in Israel and foreigner to the covenants of promise.

13 But now in Christ Jesus you who once were far away have been brought near by the blood of Christ.

14 He Himself has made two (2) one (1) and has destroyed the barrier.

15 His purpose is to create in Himself one new man out of the two, (cf. Ephesians 4:24)

18 For through Him we both have access to the Father by one

Spirit.

19 Consequently, you are no longer foreigners and aliens, but fellow citizens with God's people and members of God's household.

20 With, Christ Jesus Himself as the chief cornerstone,

21 In whom the whole building, being joined together, rises to become a holy temple in the Lord,

22 And in Him you too are being built together for a dwelling in which God by His Spirit.

What so ever there is in God is in Christ (Colossians 2:9-10; 1:19?)

Whatever there is in Christ also is in His apostles and prophets that he chose.

Whatever Paul, Peter, James and all the apostles of Jesus Christ had in them, I also have in me.

There is nothing that God put in Christ that made Him accomplish what he can read in 1 John 3:8, Acts 10:38; Acts 2:22; that God put in Peter and the Apostles that enabled then accomplish what we can see Acts 2:41, Acts 4:33; 5:12-16; Hebrews 2:4; that God put in Paul that made him do all he did as we read from scriptures

Romans 15:18:20

18 For I will not dare to speak of any of those things which Christ has not accomplished through me, in word and deed, to make the Gentiles obedient--

19 In mighty signs and wonders, by the power of the Spirit of God, so that from Jerusalem and round about to Illyricum I have fully preached the gospel of Christ.

20 And so I have made it my aim to preach the gospel, not where Christ was named, lest I should build on another man's foundation,

Acts 19:11-12

11 Now God worked unusual miracles by the hands of Paul,

12 So that even handkerchiefs or aprons were brought from his body to the sick, and the diseases left them and the evil spirits went out of them.

Acts 28:8-9

8 And it happened that the father of Publius lay sick of a fever and dysentery. Paul went in to him and prayed, and he laid his hands on him and healed him.

9 So when this was done, the rest of those on the island who had diseases also came and were healed.

2 Corinthians 12:12

Truly the signs of an apostle were accomplished among you with all perseverance, in signs and wonders and mighty deeds.

That I lack. Inside of me is conferred all each of them fore runners had in them. We are ONE New Man. Jesus Christ Made us ONE New Man a New Creature to do God works and heal all who are oppressed of the devil and stop the effects the fall, end poverty and lack in the church. As the church, we are one with Christ and have been left here to accomplished God's eternal purpose which brought Jesus Christ to this earth, and all the apostles and now, the Church.

We cannot afford to fail. We are here to fulfill God's eternal purpose of mankind's redemption and exaltation as god's upon the earth.

And we cannot fail.

We make up one family – some in heaven and some upon the earth – the whole family of God the father.

Ephesians 3:14-15

4 For this reason I bow my knees to the Father of our Lord Jesus Christ,

15 From whom the whole family in heaven and earth is named,

Ephesians 4:4 -6 (NIV)

4There is One body and One Spirit, just as you were called to one hope when you were called.

5 One Lord, One faith, one baptism;

6 One God and Father of all, who is above all, and through all, and in you all.

(See Ephesians 5:30; 1 Corinthians 6:17; Galatians 4:6-7; Ephesians 4:4-6; 2 Corinthian 6:16; Acts 10:38; Acts 2:22; John 14:12)

Do good and heal all who are oppressed by the devil and destroy all the works of the devil as Christ Jesus did and also do good and heal all and do more (greater works) than Jesus did.

CHAPTER 5

NEVER TOUCH ALL JESUS BORE AND CARRIED

Surely, He HATH BORNE our grief's (sickness) and carried our sorrows (disease)

Isaiah 53:4

Surely, He has borne our griefs and carried our sorrows; Yet we esteemed Him stricken, Smitten by God, and afflicted.

With His stripes we are healed.

Isaiah 53:5

But He was wounded for our transgressions, He was bruised for our iniquities; The chastisement for our peace was upon Him, And by His stripes we are healed.

Jesus told us that He came to fulfill the law the Prophets, not to destroy them. And He said nothing would be able to stop him until he has fulfilled all of them.

Mathew 5:17-18

17 Do not think that I came to destroy the Law or the Prophets. I did not come to destroy but to fulfill.

18 "For assuredly, I say to you, till heaven and earth pass away, one jot or one tittle will by no means pass from the law till all is fulfilled.

Shows very clearly that he fulfilled Isaiah 53:4, 5

Mathew 8:17

That it might be fulfilled which was spoken by Isaiah the prophet, saying: "He Himself took our infirmities and bore our sicknesses."

"Himself took our infirmities (diseases) and bare (carried) our sickness"

What he fulfilled must not be revisited anymore. When a matter is fulfilled, it is accomplished and matter is ended and closed. Nothing further could be done about it.

Having carried our diseases and borne our sickness, we are not to carry it anymore. We are now to hold fast the confession of our faith without wavering that we cannot be sick because he carried sickness away and we cannot be diseased because he himself took our diseases. Why must I say "I have what He carried or borne and took away from me".

To confess "I have sickness or diseases" is to make Him a liar who said He Himself took away, borne, carried off my sickness or diseases.

Instead of confessing "I have headache" say He Himself took away my headache so that I might not carry it anymore. With His stripes, I have been healed of every headache. Then thank Him for your healing.

The Living Word is our medication. Take it always by saying or speaking it.

Proverbs 4:22

For they are life to those who find them, And health to all their flesh.

Then watch out; No headache will be no more on your body. Every infirmity, sickness, grief, sorrow, disease, poverty curses etc were led on Jesus and He carried them. So I am free from them. I cannot carry them at all forever.

CHAPTER 6

PROCLAIM LIBERTY TO
THE CAPTIVES

NO ENEMY CAN HARM YOU
Jeremiah 34:1-7
1 God spoke to Jeremiah the Prophet WHEN Nebuchadnezzar king of Babylon and all his army, all the kingdoms of the earth under his dominion, and all the peoples were fighting against Jerusalem (The House or cities of the Lord) and all of its cities.

4 Yet hear the word of the LORD, O Zedekiah king of Judah! Thus says the LORD concerning you: 'You shall not die by the sword.

5 "You shall die in peace. (Psalms 91:16). For I have spoken the word, says the LORD."

6 Then Jeremiah the prophet spoke all these words to Zedekiah king of Judah in Jerusalem,

7 When the army of the king of Babylon was fighting against Jerusalem and against all the cities of Judah that were left,

No weapon formed against you shall prosper
Isaiah 54:17

No weapon formed against you shall prosper, and every tongue which rises against you in judgment You shall condemn. This is the heritage of the servants of the LORD, and their righteousness is from Me," Says the LORD.

No hair in our head can fall to the ground no matter what the enemy does (with all his host of evil and wicked forces)

To the king over God's people God says, you shall not die by the sword of the enemy and all his army or host, all his kingdom of the earth under his dominion, all his people etc fighting against you and my people. That means, regardless of the weapon he may use against you, he (the enemy) is powerless as far as your life is concerned.

The Lord has spoken the Word. It must be fulfilled.

The Word must be accomplished.

Isaiah 55:8-11

8 For My thoughts are not your thoughts, nor are your ways My ways," says the LORD.

9 For as the heavens are higher than the earth, so are My ways higher than your ways, And My thoughts than your thoughts.

10 For as the rain comes down, and the snow from heaven, and do not return there, but water the earth, and make it bring forth and bud, that it may give seed to the sower and bread to the eater,

11 So shall My word be that goes forth from My mouth; It shall not return to Me void, But it shall accomplish what I please, And it shall prosper in the thing for which I sent it.

The Word must uphold Zedekiah.

Hebrews 1:3

Who being the brightness of His glory and the express image of His person, and upholding all things by the word of His power, when He had by Himself purged our sins, sat down at the right hand of the Majesty on high,

Heaven and earth will pass away, yet the Word will not.

Mathew 5:18

For assuredly, I say to you, till heaven and earth pass away, one jot or one tittle will by no means pass from the law till all is fulfilled.

He command and it stood fast, He spoke and it was done.

Psalms 33:6, 9

6 By the word of the LORD the heavens were made, And all the host of them by the breath of His mouth.

9 For He spoke and it was done; He commanded, and it stood fast.

He will watch over His Word to perform it.

Jeremiah 1:12

Then the LORD said to me, "You have seen well, for I am ready to perform My word."

The whole world lies under wickedness.

1 John 5:19

We know that we are of God, and the whole world lies under the sway of the wicked one.

Mankind is enslaved.

Romans 8:19-22

19 For the earnest expectation of the creation eagerly waits for the revealing of the sons of God.

20 For the creation was subjected to futility, not willingly, but because of Him who subjected it in hope;

21 Because the creation itself also will be delivered from the bondage of corruption into the glorious liberty of the children of God.

22 For we know that the whole creation groans and labors with birth pangs together until now.

What are his weapons today?

Sickness, disease, war, lack, poverty, oppression, etc. Hear the Lord: You shall not die by any of these or all of them. You shall die in peace.

CHAPTER 7

There is a right way to every desired destination!

And it is following the right way only that will lead to the right destination.

God has the Right Way to your healing no matter how incurably ill you may be presently.

It is written in Proverbs 14:12 "There is a way that seems right to a man, but its end is the way of death."

Let's look at the way to healing that appeared right to people in Scriptures that led to their suffering, poetry or death.

1 Asa died because he sought physicians and not the Lord:

II Chronicles 16:12-13

12 And in the thirty-ninth year of his reign, Asa became diseased in his feet, and his malady was severe; yet in his disease he did not seek the LORD, but the physicians.

13 So Asa rested with his fathers; he died in the forty-first year of his reign.

2. The woman suffered at the hands of physicians

Mark 5:26

And had suffered many things from many physicians. She had spent all that she had and was no better, but rather grew worse.

3 The woman spent all she had and was made poor by phys-

icians through medical bills.

Mark 5:26

And had suffered many things from many physicians. She had spent all that she had and was no better, but rather grew worse.

4 Physicians could not heal the woman of her sickness.

Luke 8:43

Now a woman, having a flow of blood for twelve years, who had spent all her livelihood on physicians and could not be healed by any,

5. Job after his encounters with his doctors and suffering called all his doctors "forgers of lies and Worthless Physicians."

Job 13:4 "But you forgers of lies, you are all worthless physicians."

6. King Ahaziah died for going to consult the god of Ekron when he was sick

2Kings 1:2-4,16-17

2 Now Ahaziah fell through the lattice of his upper room in Samaria, and was injured; so, he sent messengers and said to them, "Go, inquire of Baal-Zebub, the god of Ekron, whether I shall recover from this injury."

3 But the angel of the LORD said to Elijah the Tishbite, "Arise, go up to meet the messengers of the king of Samaria, and say to them, 'Is it because there is no God in Israel that you are going to inquire of Baal-Zebub, the god of Ekron?'

4 "Now therefore, thus says the LORD: 'You shall not come down from the bed to which you have gone up, but you shall surely die.'"

16 Then he said to him, "Thus says the LORD: 'Because you have sent messengers to inquire of Baal-Zebub, the god of Ekron, is it because there is no God in Israel to inquire of His word? Therefore, you shall not come down from the bed to which you have gone up, but you shall surely die.'"

17 So Ahaziah died according to the word of the LORD which Elijah had spoken.

Did you notice that Luke the beloved Physicians never wrote anything about himself to show he practiced administering

drugs or medicine to the sick?

Read Luke's gospel and the Acts of the Apostles and you will not find a verse of Scripture he wrote to uphold medicine in dealing with the problem of sickness and disease.

Doctor Luke wrote to show the supremacy of The Living Word of God and the Divine Ways of God in healing the sick of all sicknesses and diseases over man's method or medicine. See Acts 19:11-12; Acts 28 1-10; Acts 5:12-16.

Colossians 4:14 says Luke the beloved physician and Demas greet you. I like the name Paul called Luke by the Holy Spirit. "Luke the Beloved Physician!"

Scriptures show that the sick need the Physician and Jesus is the Physician.

Luke 5:31

Jesus answered and said to them, "Those who are well have no need of a physician, but those who are sick.

Mark 2:17

When Jesus heard it, He said to them, "Those who are well have no need of a physician, but those who are sick. I did not come to call the righteous, but sinners, to repentance."

Mathew 9:12

When Jesus heard that, He said to them, "Those who are well have no need of a physician, but those who are sick.

Exodus 15:26

And said, "If you diligently heed the voice of the LORD your God and do what is right in His sight, give ear to His commandments and keep all His statutes, I will put none of the diseases on you which I have brought on the Egyptians. For I am the LORD who heals you."

Acts 10:38

How God anointed Jesus of Nazareth with the Holy Spirit and with power, who went about doing good and healing all who were oppressed by the devil, for God was with Him.

8 There is a Balm in Gilead (Hill of witness or Zion – The Church)

Mathew 18:19-20

19 Again I say to you that if two of you agree on earth concerning anything that they ask, it will be done for them by My Father in heaven.

20 For where two or three are gathered together in My name, I am there in the midst of them."

Where we gather, Jesus is there – and is there to heal. The Church –Body of Christ is the Healing center of the LORD. There is the presence of the Physicians (the Healer) with His Anointing to heal and deliver.

Everyone is to come to the healing center and be healed (John 8:19B)

Isaiah 2:2-3

2 Now it shall come to pass in the latter days That the mountain of the LORD'S house Shall be established on the top of the mountains, and shall be exalted above the hills; And all nations shall flow to it.

3 Many people shall come and say, "Come, and let us go up to the mountain of the LORD, To the house of the God of Jacob; He will teach us His ways, and we shall walk in His paths." For out of Zion shall go forth the law, And the word of the LORD from Jerusalem.

Micah 4:1-2

1 Now it shall come to pass in the latter days That the mountain of the LORD'S house Shall be established on the top of the mountains, and shall be exalted above the hills; And peoples shall flow to it.

2 Many nations shall come and say, "Come, and let us go up to the mountain of the LORD, To the house of the God of Jacob; He will teach us His ways, and we shall walk in His paths." For out of Zion the law shall go forth, And the word of the LORD from Jerusalem.

Bring all of the sick into the Hill of witness (Gilead or the Church or Mount Zion) and the Great Physicians will settle all their cases.

Luke 14:21-23

21 So that servant came and reported these things to his master. Then the master of the house, being angry, said to his ser-

vant, 'Go out quickly into the streets and lanes of the city, and bring in here the poor and the maimed and the lame and the blind.'

22 And the servant said, 'Master, it is done as you commanded, and still there is room.'

23 Then the master said to the servant, 'Go out into the highways and hedges, and compel them to come in, that my house may be filled.

Mathew 21:12-14

12 Then Jesus went into the temple of God and drove out all those who bought and sold in the temple, and overturned the tables of the money changers and the seats of those who sold doves.

13 And He said to them, "It is written, 'My house shall be called a house of prayer,' but you have made it a 'den of thieves.'"

14 Then the blind and the lame came to Him in the temple, and He healed them.

"Is the Lord not in Zion?

"Is her King not in her?

Jeremiah 8:19

19 Listen! The voice, the cry of the daughter of my people from a far country: "Is not the LORD in Zion? Is not her King in her?" "Why have they provoked Me to anger with their carved images- With foreign idols?"

There is a balm for the healing of all manner of sickness or disease in Gilead – Hill of witness or Zion.

You only need to come and be healed. Giving elsewhere is simply to allow yourself be destroyed.

CHAPTER 8

THE DOOR TO THE MIRACULOUS

Healing: speaking opens the door to the miraculous
Luke 16:16 (RSV)
The law and the prophets were until John; since then the good news of the kingdom of God is preached, and every one enters it violently. (cf. Mathew 11:12-13)

To preach is to proclaim or declare. The gospel in the power of God (Romans 1:16). That means until the power of God, the ability of God is proclaimed or declared, the way of entrance remains shut and none can be able to enter.

It is therefore, the proclamation of the word or power of God that open the door and paves the way for everyone to enter violently.

If people must enter the kingdom of God, then first of all, we must preach or declare or proclaim the Word or power of God to them that are outside.

We say boldly what we believe. The Spirit of faith is simply declaring what we believe regardless of the circumstances
2 Corinthians 4:13
And since we have the same spirit of faith, according to what is written, "I believed and therefore I spoke," we also believe and therefore speak,
The word I speak to you is Spirit and life. The Spirit of faith = to

the word of faith.

John 6:63

It is the Spirit who gives life; the flesh profits nothing. The words that I speak to you are spirit, and they are life.

By faith, we quench or stop all the fiery darts of the enemy's arrows (Ephesians 6:16)

Luke 21:15

For I will give you a mouth and wisdom which all your adversaries will not be able to contradict or resist.

When we speak by faith all we believe, the spirit of faith goes into work to birth what the word of faith we speak desires. When God said "let there be", the spirit of faith caused what God said to materialize. By the Spirit of faith, the word of faith we believe and speak materializes in living proofs.

The Spirit of faith is God's cure to the Spirit of fear but can only work when believers begin to boldly say what the word of God says. We must believe and speak if what we desire to be done is to be done,

We believe and so we speak.

We don't wait to see before we speak

We don't wait to see before we believe.

We disallow circumstances from keeping us from speaking

We speak boldly what we believe to happen, not what we see, hear, touch, taste or smell to be happening.

It is our commitment to be speaking what we believe to happen that will out the Spirit of faith (2 Corinthians 4:13) to work to cause the word of faith (Romans 10:8) to produce the works of faith (James 2:13:14-26)

Whatever we want to see, believe to see, we spoke and He saw.

Whatever we want to see, Believe, then speak and you will see it. Preaching the gospel is to proclaim The Living Word. It is what opens the door to the MIRACULOUS and manifests same anywhere. Proclaiming The Living Word open the prison doors and releases the captives.

Jesus taught the people and proclaimed the gospel and the results were the things He did which the people saw.

Luke 20:1-2

1 Now it happened on one of those days, as He taught the people in the temple and preached the gospel, that the chief priests and the scribes, together with the elders, confronted Him

2 and spoke to Him, saying, "Tell us, by what authority are You doing these things? Or who is he who gave You this authority?"

Proclaimed the word opens the way to signs and wonders and miraculous.

Luke 4:18-19

18 The Spirit of the LORD is upon Me, Because He has anointed Me To preach the gospel to the poor; He has sent Me to heal the brokenhearted, to proclaim liberty to the captives and recovery of sight to the blind, to set at liberty those who are oppressed;

19 To proclaim the acceptable year of the LORD."

Isaiah 61:1-4

1 The Spirit of the Lord GOD is upon Me, Because the LORD has anointed Me To preach good tidings to the poor; He has sent Me to heal the brokenhearted, To proclaim liberty to the captives, And the opening of the prison to those who are bound;

2 To proclaim the acceptable year of the LORD, And the day of vengeance of our God; To comfort all who mourn,

3 To console those who mourn in Zion, To give them beauty for ashes, The oil of joy for mourning, The garment of praise for the spirit of heaviness; That they may be called trees of righteousness, The planting of the LORD, that He may be glorified."

4 And they shall rebuild the old ruins, they shall raise up the former desolations, and they shall repair the ruined cities, The desolations of many generations.

Preaching the gospel or proclaiming the word (power) of God always resulted in indescribable miracles.

Luke 4:40-44

40 When the sun was setting, all those who had any that were sick with various diseases brought them to Him; and He laid His hands on every one of them and healed them.

41 And demons also came out of many, crying out and saying, "You are the Christ, the Son of God!" And He, rebuking them, did

not allow them to speak, for they knew that He was the Christ.

42 Now when it was day, He departed and went into a deserted place. And the crowd sought Him and came to Him, and tried to keep Him from leaving them;

43 But He said to them, "I must preach the kingdom of God to the other cities also, because for this purpose I have been sent."

44 And He was preaching in the synagogues of Galilee.

Mathew 4:23-25

23 And Jesus went about all Galilee, teaching in their synagogues, preaching the gospel of the kingdom, and healing all kinds of sickness and all kinds of disease among the people.

24 Then His fame went throughout all Syria; and they brought to Him all sick people who were afflicted with various diseases and torments, and those who were demon-possessed, epileptics, and paralytics; and He healed them.

25 Great multitudes followed Him--from Galilee, and from Decapolis, Jerusalem, Judea, and beyond the Jordan.

Mathew 9:35-38

35 Then Jesus went about all the cities and villages, teaching in their synagogues, preaching the gospel of the kingdom, and healing every sickness and every disease among the people.

36 But when He saw the multitudes, He was moved with compassion for them, because they were weary and scattered, like sheep having no shepherd.

37 Then He said to His disciples, "The harvest truly is plentiful, but the laborers are few.

38 Therefore pray the Lord of the harvest to send out laborers into His harvest."

Proclaim what God is doing, has done and you will see the same happen.

The people cannot be free until they hear what God has done, is doing and can do. This is the whole essence of preaching.

The spirit of faith must be expressed through the word of faith to birth the works.

TESTIMONY OF HEALING TODAY

A LUMP ON MY WIFE'S ABDOMEN DESTROYED

My wife had a serious attack this morning as she woke up at about 2.00am. She could not sleep again till about 4:49 when I woke up. She told me what happened. And I laid my hands on her and commanded that evil spirit to get out and for every pain to cease. I touched her abdomen and behold, there was a big lump. That was an oppression of the devil. I took my anointing oil, anointed it and commanded that lump to dissolve and disappear in Jesus Name. Instantly, that big lump dissolved and disappeared to the glory of God. I just give God All the Glory.

I remember reading testimonies of people who had growth(s) in them that they spent fortunes to get them out with the knives of medical doctors all to no avail. But for me, God did it, without any charge. Father I just thank you for your faithfulness to us in Jesus Name.

CHAPTER 9

It is written "You will show me the path of life; In Your presence is fullness of joy; At Your right hand are pleasures forevermore." Psalm 16:11

GOD'S ORDAINED WAY TO A HEALTHY LIFE

Psalm 103:2-5

2 Bless the LORD, O my soul, and forget not all His benefits:

3 Who forgives all your iniquities, who heals all your diseases,

4 Who redeems your life from destruction, who crowns you with lovingkindness and tender mercies,

5 Who satisfies your mouth with good things, so that your youth is renewed like the eagle's.

Common sense to a healthy life

1.Health and food: You Are What You Eat

Benjamin Franklin says "We should eat to live and not live to eat" Mind what you eat, when you eat, why you eat, what you eat, hoe you eat, with whom you eat, where you eat, food for the body and body for the food but both God shall destroy. Avoid fat, salt, prepared canned / tinned food.

2. Dietary Control and Cancer

High fat foods are a problem. Meat consumption causes colon cancer.

Depend on plant foods, vegetables, fruits, legumes, grains, fish and dairy products (milk) moderately, honey, bread. You may work to take a little of meat, poultry, fish dairy products; But never depend on them nor make them a part of your daily meal.

Live on vegetables, plant foods, legumes, fruits, grains, honey and fruits.

Fruits and vegetables prevent heart diseases, cancer, obesity and excess weight and its attendant diseases.

3. Exercise for your health

1Timothy 4:8

For bodily exercise profits a little, but godliness is profitable for all things, having promise of the life that now is and of that which is to come.

"There is solid evidence that physically active people live longer ....

Fitness helped overcome all causes of mortality, including diabetes, cancer, and heart diseases" (Kenneth H. Cooper M.D, It's Better to Believe, 1995, p 211)

"Regular physical activity reduces the risk for developing or dying from coronary heart disease, noninsulin dependent diabetes, hypertension, and colon cancer reduces symptoms of anxiety and depression; contribute to the development and maintenance of healthier bones, muscles and joints and helps control weight "(The surgeon general of United States report in "Morbidity and Mortality Weekly Report, July 12, 1996, p.591)

Always Endeavour to exercise. It must not be vigorous to be beneficial. Walk. Work in your garden. Enjoy in physical activity.

Man's deterioration is as a result of decreased effectiveness of heart and lungs. Frequent, regular, physical exercise checks this deterioration, slows and even reverses the deterioration. Running, jogging, cycling, swimming, walking out at health clubs, homes exercise machines / devices etc are important.

Exercise and Reduced fat intake checks weight.

4. Sleep is Time to Recharge

Sufficient sleep is essential to good health. God giveth his beloved sleep (Psalms 127:1-2)

Most people can't sleep. They have a very serious problem with their health.

In 1977, there were 3 certified sleep clinics in America and by 1997 the number had grown to 337 (Making Life Work, Page 25 – Key to a Healthy, Long Life)

The US Department of Transport "estimates that sleepy drivers cause at least 56, 000 accidents every year" (America) medical News, July 17, 1995)

Sleep loss reduces the body resistance to disease, sickness and infections. Insomnia is a disease. It causes "difficulty is falling asleep or remaining asleep" for all suffering from this disease, there is healing. You will sleep very soundly from now.

Bodily exercise enhances our ability to get sound, restful sleep. Evidence of intake for stimulants of caffeine, nicotine etc is a must. Try ceasing your work or intense mental exercise / activity I hour before you go to bed. Try keeping regular home for going to bed and getting up. Take a warm bath before bedtime. It induces sleep, too.

Sleep helps restore our bodies and minds. God works when we sleep.

5. Take care to Avoid Injury

Accidents are available. It takes being divinely led and guided by God's Holy Spirit. In 1997, 41, 967 died and 3.4 million were injured in USE. In Nigeria, the record can only be imagined.

Most of these accidents could be prevented with caution and safe driving habits.

6. Avoid the Use of Dangerous Substances

Drugs, tobacco, liquor etc.

"The global proliferation of cigarettes leads to an estimated 3 million death a year... By 2020, the number is estimated by the world Health Organization, to reach 10 million a year" (Cart Sagan, Billion and Billions, 1997, p 205)

Take a random sample of a thousand young men who smoke on the basis of actuarial data it can confidently be predicted that one of these young men will eventually be murdered, six will be killed on the roads and 250 will die prematurely from the effects of smoking (Martin P.59)

Tobacco is a deadly substance. Its smoke "contains more than 4000 chemicals including trace amounts of such known poisons as cyanide, arsenic, and formaldehyde. There are 43 known cancer – causing chemicals (carcinogens) in tobacco smokes "(Mayo Clinic Family Health Book, 1996, P317).

Tobacco users are very highly susceptible to numerous diseases of a variety of cancers, cardiovascular ailments, sexual dysfunction and lung diseases, including emphysema.

"Each year smoking kills more than 400,000 Americans more than died in battle in world war 11 and the victim's war combined "(Mayo Clinic Family Health Book, 1996, P 316).

7.We must honour and glorify God in our bodies

1 Corinthians 6:20

For you were bought at a price; therefore, glorify God in your body and in your spirit, which are God's.

Exodus 20:3

You shall have no other gods before Me.

Romans 6:16

Do you not know that to whom you present yourselves slaves to obey, you are that one's slaves whom you obey, whether of sin leading to death, or of obedience leading to righteousness?

Mathew 4:10

Then Jesus said to him, "Away with you, Satan! For it is written, 'You shall worship the LORD your God, and Him only you shall serve.'"

Don't be enslaved. Serve God wholly.

Alcohol is the 3rd – largest in the USA ranking before heart disease (1st) and cancer (2nd). Alcohol damages the brain, nerves, liver, pancreas and cardiovascular system. Alcoholism causes cancer.

"After cardiovascular disease, cancer is the next leading. Cause of death among alcoholics "(Mayo Clinic Family Health Book, P 329).

Avoid alcohol (See Proverbs 20:1, Proverbs 23:1; Ephesians 5:18. 1; 1 Corinthians 6:10)

8. The Power of a Positive Outlook

Positive thought and emotions help promote physical health.

Negative thought and emotions affect health of individuals.

Many Cardiac patients' medical researchers have shown tended to be competitive, impatient and always in a hurry. They always end up with coronary disease.

"Hostility and Cynicism" are the real risk factors for heart disease (News week), Feb. 17, 1997)

Stress, negative emotions example anxiety and depression causes health hazards examples cold and cancer.

9. Positive emotion boost health

Proverbs 17:22

A merry heart does good, like medicine, but a broken spirit dries the bones.

Proverbs 18:14

The spirit of a man will sustain him in sickness, but who can bear a broken spirit?

10. Marriage promotes life and health

I. It is not good for man to be alone

Genesis 2:18

And the LORD God said, "It is not good that man should be alone; I will make him a helper comparable to him."

II. Woe to him that is alone

Ecclesiastes 4:9-12

9 Two are better than one, because they have a good reward for their labor.

10 For if they fall, one will lift up his companion. But woe to him who is alone when he falls, for he has no one to help him up.

11 Again, if two lie down together, they will keep warm; But how can one be warm alone?

12 Though one may be overpowered by another, two can withstand him. And a threefold cord is not quickly broken.

III. Male and Female crated He them and Blessed them.

Genesis 1:27-28

27 So God created man in His own image; in the image of God He created him; male and female He created them.

28 Then God blessed them, and God said to them, "Be fruitful and multiply; fill the earth and subdue it; have dominion over the fish of the sea, over the birds of the air, and over every living thing that moves on the earth."

11. People need people to stay healthy (Hebrews 10:25; Psalms 133:1-3; Mathew 18:16-20; Ecclesiastes 4:8-12)

12. Love is the greatest.

God is Love and Health personified.

God Loves and Gives! Love is giving to another, not to yourself, what will make the other the best.

The nourishment of relationships, both with God and with our fellowmen, is a proven health principle.

13. Take personal responsibility for your health

3 John 2

I wish above all things that thou (you) mayest prosper and be in health, even as thy (your) soul prospereth.

14. Healthy people share one of life's greatest blessings – Their lives with others.

Don't abuse one of the greatest treasures God has given to you. Observe health rules and live long to serve God, man and yourself.

This is one of the greatest secret to a healthy living. When you sow your life as a seed, and allow it to die, it reproduces many other lives.

Luke 14:25-27 "Now great multitudes went with Him. And He turned and said to them, If anyone comes to Me and does not hate his father and mother, wife and children, brothers and sisters, yes, and his own life also, he cannot be My disciple. And whoever does not bear his cross and come after Me cannot be My disciple."

Luke 9:23-24 "Then He said to them all, "If anyone desires to come after Me, let him deny himself, and take up his cross daily, and follow Me. For whoever desires to save his life will lose it, but whoever loses his life for My sake will save it."

John 12:23-26 says "But Jesus answered them, saying, "The hour has come that the Son of Man should be glorified. Most assuredly, I say to you, unless a grain of wheat falls into the ground and dies, it remains alone; but if it dies, it produces much grain. He who loves his life will lose it, and he who hates his life in this world will keep it for eternal life. If anyone serves Me, let him follow Me; and where I am, there My servant will be also. If anyone serves Me, him My Father will honor."

God's most profound ordained way to a healthy Life is for you to Share your life by planting it as a seed to serve others and you will have it given back to you as your harvest supernaturally blessed and preserved blameless, spirit, soul and body with many other lives,

Begin to live for others from this day and you will enjoy a healthy life.

God bless you. Peace!

BECOME A CITIZEN OF HEAVEN TODAY!

Please note, if you are not yet a Citizen of Heaven, but desire to be, this is your opportunity. To be a citizen of Heaven, you must be from above. You must be born of God. You must be born again!

John 3:3-8,12-13

3 Jesus answered and said to him, "Most assuredly, I say to you, unless one is born again, he cannot see the kingdom of God."

4 Nicodemus said to Him, "How can a man be born when he is old? Can he enter a second time into his mother's womb and be born?"

5 Jesus answered, "Most assuredly, I say to you, unless one is born of water and the Spirit, he cannot enter the kingdom of God.

6 "That which is born of the flesh is flesh, and that which is born of the Spirit is spirit.

7 "Do not marvel that I said to you, 'You must be born again.'

8 "The wind blows where it wishes, and you hear the sound of it, but cannot tell where it comes from and where it goes. So is everyone who is born of the Spirit."

12 If I have told you earthly things, and ye believe not, how shall ye believe, if I tell you of heavenly things?

13 And no man hath ascended up to heaven, but he that came down from heaven, even the Son of man which is in heaven.

Jesus says "You must be born again to live and enjoy Heaven-now!" John 3:3,7

No matter your sin(s) and what you may have done, God wants you forgive and restored now!

John 3:13-18

13 "No one has ascended to heaven but He who came down from heaven, that is, the Son of Man who is in heaven.

14 "And as Moses lifted up the serpent in the wilderness, even so must the Son of Man be lifted up,

15 "that whoever believes in Him should not perish but have eternal life.

16 "For God so loved the world that He gave His only begotten Son, that whoever believes in Him should not perish but have everlasting life.

17 "For God did not send His Son into the world to condemn the world, but that the world through Him might be saved.

18 "He who believes in Him is not condemned; but he who does not believe is condemned already, because he has not believed in the name of the only begotten Son of God.

Remember God gives the power to become His son to everyone that receives Jesus as The Christ, The Son of The Living God or believe in His Name. John 1:12

Remember God Himself dwells in everyone who believes and confesses that Jesus is The Christ, The Son of The Living God. 1John 5:1, 4-5;1John 4:4,15

Remember God did not send His Son into the world to condemn the world but that through Him, the world might be saved. John 3:17

Beloved, AS the Father sent Jesus The Christ, even so has The Lord Jesus Christ sent me so that everyone who will believe and receive me as His Ambassador will be saved, healed, delivered and restored. The Lord said to me: As the Father sent Me, even so have I sent you! John 17:18; John 20:21

The Lord said to Me: Verily, verily I say to you, whoever receives you receives me, and whoever receives me receives the Father who sent me. John 13:20.

The Lord said to Me: Whoever rejects you rejects me, and whoever rejects Me rejects The Father who sent Me. Luke 10:16

The Lord said to Me: Behold I give unto you power to tread upon serpents and scorpions and over all the power of the enemy and nothing shall by any means hurt you. Luke 10:19

The Lord said to Me: Behold, I send in the midst of many peoples, like dew from the LORD, like showers on the grass, that tarry for no man nor wait for the sons of men. Behold, you shall be among the Gentiles, In the midst of many peoples, like a lion among the beasts of the forest, like a young lion among flocks of sheep, Who, if he passes through, both treads down and tears in pieces, and none can deliver. Your hand shall be lifted against your adversaries, and all your enemies shall be cut off. Micah 5:7-9

The Lord said to Me: You will be like the dew to all My people and creation; You shall grow like the lily, and lengthen Your roots like Lebanon. Your branches shall spread; Your beauty shall be like an olive tree, And Your fragrance like Lebanon. Those who dwell under Your shadow shall return; They shall be revived like grain, and grow like a vine. Their scent shall be like the wine of Lebanon. Hosea 14:5-7

Beloved, there is no justifiable reason under Heaven why you should ever go through ANYTHING that is not in Heaven now!

Beloved there is no justifiable reason why you should not have NOW the best God has fully paid for and credited to your personal account!

Hear Me: All things are ready. And all things are yours! What are you still waiting for? All you need to do is to believe that Jesus is the Christ, The Son of The Living God. And He sent Me to bring this Goodnews to you.

Your struggles can come to an end today. You can be enrolled into Heaven's citizenship right now. You can begin a new life today and enjoy all that is available in Heaven from this day forward. The Lord Jesus Christ who sent me confirms with undeniable proof that He is ALIVE today in the lives of those who hear my words and believes in Him [The Lord Jesus Christ] who sent me.

Jesus is alive today and the only way to prove it is for Him to do what He did before in your life today. He sent me and will prove to you that this is not a made-up story written to impress you, but His ordained will made available to make you are created to be!

The choice is yours! Rise and take what belong to you and enter your rest!

Peace now and always in Jesus Almighty Name!

Amen!!!

If You are not certain that You are Born Again as you are certain of your name, or You were once saved but went astray again, living and doing as you pleased, then say this Prayer aloud now for you to become a citizen of Heaven:

PRAYER FOR SALVATION AND RESTORATION TO HEAVEN'S CITIZENSHIP!

Dear Heavenly Father, I return to you by Faith. I am sorry for my sins. I believe in my heart that Jesus is The Christ and that He died for my sins and rose from the dead on the third day, according to Scripture, for my justification. I confess that Jesus Christ is LORD and I accept Him now as my Saviour. I believe my sins are wiped away.

I call upon The Name of The LORD for my total Healing, Liberty and Restoration.

I ask for the Gift of Your Holy Spirit, Power and Grace to follow and serve You from this day forward. And I Thank You Abba Father for doing far beyond all I have asked and can ever imagine in Jesus Name. Amen!

I Now Declare That I Am A Child of God Forever! There's no going back.

Now that you have become a Citizen of Heaven, you need to upgrade by signing up to serve as an Ambassador for Christ. That is where your security and relevance lie. There is no job in this world that can be compared to serving as The Ambassador of The King of kings and Lord of lords. The benefits are amazing. You cannot do a better or more honourable job.

You can Enlist now and become a Partner or a Member of

our Totally Empowered Ambassadors on Mission (TEAM) and see what Our Risen Lord and King Jesus Christ will transform your life into and do in, for and through you from this day as you believe and obey His Word!

I can't wait to hear from you because I believe you have been blessed and helped immensely reading this Book as much as I am writing it! I am praying for you.

ABOUT THE AUTHOR

Amb. Promise Ogbonna

Amb Promise Ogbonna is the President of Christ's Ambassadors Living Mission International Inc. aka Jesus Mission Headquarters, an all-encompassing network of ministries with a mandate focus to Preach The Everlasting Gospel to all, Stop anything after man's destruction, Bring Healing, Liberty and Restoration to all, Make ALL Christ's Ambassadors and Make Heaven-Now a Reality for All.

He is the Publisher of ONTOP Life Publishers Company with a commission to Publish the Everlasting Gospel and Bring God's Wisdom-solutions for every problem and need of mankind.

He represents The Lord Jesus Christ and serves Him as His Ambassador!

He is married and blessed with children.

OTHER BOOKS BY AMB PROMISE OGBONNA

1. The Nothingness of Satan
2. You Can Make a Fresh Start and Rule Your World
3. Restoring the Forgotten Dignity of Woman
4. Christ's Ambassadors: Re-Emergence of Rulers in
5. Why Prophet Elisha Died Sick and how to Avoid it
6. You Can Choose When to Die
7. You Shall Live and Not Die
8. Why Christians Die Sick
9. 7 Keys to Undeniable Healing
10. 8 Decisive Hours That Will Take You to The Topmost
11. Activating God's Medicine for Your Healing
12. God Cannot Fail to Heal You
13. Healing Is Your Legal Right
14. God's Final Solution to The Problem of The Black Race
15. Understanding God's Secret to Winning Life's Battles
16. 100 Years Is Minimum
17. How to Raise the Dead
18. Manifesting ss Signs and Wonders: Unlocking the Unstoppable You Regardless of Where You are Now!
19. 40 Pitfalls to Avoid in Life – Mastering the Art of Living Successfully.
20. Wisdom Seeds to Greatness in Life – Inspiring Seed-Thoughts on Being Your Best
21. God's Medicine for Incurable Diseases
22. Ambassador Promise: Jesus Christ's Official Ambassador and T. L. Osborn's Successor on Earth Today! Appearance and En-

counters with The Lord Jesus Christ, Mantles of Notable Servants of God Received and the 9 Mandates.

23. Simple Faith for Supernatural Success
24. God's Final Message to The Poor
25. Understanding the Gospel to The Poor
26. Faith That Attracts God's Attention and Results
27. God's Quickest Way to Your Prosperity and Restoration
28. Faith for Healing
29. Unveiling God's Master Keys to Your Dominion Against All Odds
30. Operating the Faith that Pleases God
31. 4 Kinds of People the Lord Will Heal
32. Appropriating Your Healing
33. Why Divine Healing
34. Secrets to Making Your Faith Work
35. The Right Use of The Anointing Oil
36. Healing All Manner of Sicknesses & Diseases
37. Christ's Ambassadors Handbook: Volume 1
38. Christ's Ambassadors Handbook: Volume 2
39. Christ's Ambassadors Handbook: Volume 3
40. God's Secret to Wealth and Health
41. Enforcing Your Covenant of Divine Health
42. Faith for Miracles
43. Christ's Teaching on God's Secret to Kingdom Prosperity
44. The Prerequisite for Doing God's Will and Finishing His Work
45. The Wonders of The New Creation
46. Secrets of Being A Relevant Shepherd & Minister of Christ
47. Will the Lord Heal All Today?
48. Jesus Christ heals All The Sick Today!
49. God Will Heal Even The Worst Sinners Of Any Sickness

UPCOMING BOOKS BY AMB PROMISE OGBONNA

1. Enforcing Kingdom Wealth Transfer
2. God's Final Word on Tithes, Tithing and Offerings
3. Creating Heaven Out of Your Ruined World
4. How to Attract God's Blessing on Your Business and Career
5. God's Master Key to Your Dominion
6. Wisdom Keys to God's Recovery Plan
7. Why People Fail in Life –Secrets to Success without Stress

Please visit your favorite eBook retailer to discover other books by Amb Promise Ogbonna.

CONNECT WITH AMB PROMISE OGBONNA

I appreciate you reading my book. Here are my links and Social Coordinates

Send Amb Promise Ogbonna a mail at:

Visit Amb. Promise Ogbonna's Website:

Subscribe to Amb Promise Ogbonna's videos at:

Follow Amb Promise Ogbonna on Twitter:

Friend Amb Promise Ogbonna on Facebook:

Connect with Amb Promise Ogbonna on LinkedIn:

Read Amb Promise Ogbonna's Story at Wattpad:

Subscribe to Amb Promise Ogbonna's Blog at:

Follow Amb Promise Ogbonna on Instagram:

Subscribe to Amb. Promise Ogbonna's HEAVENow You Tube Channel:

Read Amb Promise Ogbonna's Smashwords Interview at

Read Amb Promise Ogbonna's Author Profile at Smashwords:

Follow Amb Promise Ogbonna at Amazon:

Connect with Amb Promise Ogbonna on Pinterest:

Read Amb. Promise Ogbonna books at Okada Books:

Get Access to all the Books of Amb Promise Ogbonna at Books2Read Universal Book Link:

Join Amb. Promise Ogbonna
in HEAVENow Services

Worship with Ambassador Promise in Christ's Ambassadors Heaven-Now Services at:
Christ's Ambassadors Living Mission International [Jesus Mission Headquarters]

24 Independence Street, Behind O'Mark Schools by O'Mark Bus Stop, LASU Road, Igando Lagos

Wednesdays: 12:00-1:00pm. Hour of EmPowerment for All [Online]

Saturdays: 8:00-9:00am. Hour of Healing for All

Sundays: 8:00-9:00am. Hour of Liberty and Restoration for All

Sundays: 9:00-10:00am. Hour of Kingdom Wealth Transfer for All

Last Friday Night Monthly: 10pm. Night of Restorations for All

Ambassadors International Bible Institute: Runs Online and Offline Courses to Make Christ's Ambassadors and Make Heaven Now a reality for all. Enroll today!

HEAVENow...Making Heaven now a Reality for ALL!

OUR HEALING PRODUCTS

We are on a Mission to Bring Healing to the sick no matter their sicknesses or diseases and Restore Health, Wealth and Peace to ALL! Here are some of our Products and Services we run to Bring Healing to the sick worldwide!

1. All-Purpose Divine Healing Medicine
2. Healing Messages – Podcasts, CD, MP3 and DVD
3. Healing Books
4. Healing Leaves Magazine
5. Healing Anointing Oil
6. Healing Mantles and Clothes
7. Healing Materials
8. Healing Elixir for incurable diseases
9. Healing Songs
10. Healing Homes
11. Health Centers
12. Healing Balm

Call us today for all of your Healing needs! We are here to SERVE YOU!

For Bookings Contact Amb Promise Ogbonna at: ambpromiseogbonna@gmail.com or Call +234 8060638053

OUR SPECIAL SERVICES

We Offer the following services to Churches, Ministries, Corporate Bodies, Businesses, Communities, Groups, International Bodies, NGO's, Governments, States and Nations.

1. Healing Seminars
2. Healing School
3. Healing Teams
4. Healing Outreaches and Explosions
5. World Healing Conferences
6. Health and Wealth Trainings
7. Heaven-Now Campaigns
8. Kingdom Wealth Transfer Seminars
9. God's FASTEST Prosperity Recovery Seminars
10. Heaven's Business School
11. Time and Stress Management Training
12. Leadership Responsibility Development Training

Our Services are geared towards making every person fit spirit, soul and body so that they can be empowered to deliver results competently, effectively and efficiently.

For Bookings Contact Amb Promise Ogbonna at: ambpromiseogbonna@gmail.com or Call +234 8060638053